The Truth About Longevity In Good Health

"If we could give every individual the right amount of nourishment and exercise, not too little and not too much, we would have found the safest way to health."

— Hippocrates

Table of contents

Introduction

Longevity is defined in the dictionary as 'the long duration of an individual life'. Quite naturally, most people wish to live as long a life as possible and aim for longevity, that is, living longer than the average.

The aim of this book is to look at various factors which contribute to the longevity (or otherwise) of human life and to provide you with all the information you need about the positive steps one can take to live a long, happy and healthy life.

Whilst we will examine age related trends amongst the world population, biological influences and research, the emphasis of this book is on the role that food can play in our health. Don't worry, this is not about dieting or simply eating less, it focuses on the categories and types of food that can bring you wonderful health benefits. Most importantly, the book will let you know which to avoid and why, so that, with a few simple changes in lifestyle, you can have a positive and long lasting impact on your own longevity.

Longevity

Thanks to modern medicine, its rapid developments and continual research, it has resulted in more information being available than ever before about the various factors which affect our health and well-being. The changes to life expectancy over the last 150 years or so have been nothing short of staggering. Just imagine, a baby born in 1900 was expected to live about 50 years, now the life expectancy of people in the United States is nearly 79 years on average, a remarkable increase, but should an average person's longevity be even higher? Given the eradication of certain diseases that would previously have been fateful, improved sanitation and hygiene in the developed world, the answer is almost certainly yes.

What Determines Your Longevity?

Suprisingly, whilst many people assume that longevity is 'all in the genes' they actually only account for around 30% of your life expectancy. The remaining 70% is the result how you behave ie the choices you make, attitudes, your environment and a small amount of good fortune.

Clearly nobody wants to die sooner than they have to. You want to live a life where you are able to see your kids, even grandkids, graduate high school, graduate college, get married and create beautiful wonderful families of their own, which you can engage in and enjoy for the rest of your life. Sometimes though you make small choices, choices which you don't realise can alter the entire trajectory of your life moving forward. Let's start by talking about our DNA.

There are many theories about aging, but what research has shown is that there are three important parts of the DNA which control aging and longevity. Most of our DNA codes for proteins, but these three enzymes change how the DNA responds to our environment in terms of longevity and aging. They don't control or create new proteins. They tell the rest of our genes and the rest of our DNA, what to do.

There are two pathways when it comes to every cell in the body: growth and reproduction, or protection and maintenance. Growth and reproduction means that cells are replicating again and again to create new cells. With protection and maintenance, the cells are not replicating, reproducing, nor growing. They're just maintaining the status quo. The three enzymes we're going to talk about are responsible for which pathway a cell takes, and thus whether it ages or stays young.

Centenarian Populations around the World

People who reach the age of 100 years or more, are currently the fastest growing part of the population. You have learned a little about where they live, how they live, and have taken away maybe one or two of their secrets. So you may now be wondering just how many centenarians are there currently living on this planet we call home? Current estimates put the figure of total centenarians worldwide at about 450,000. Exact numbers may be difficult to determine, since many centenarians live in developing or outlying areas, where census data is not often available. However, the number of centenarians in industrialized nations is still rather impressive.

The West

In total numbers the United States has the most centenarians with current estimates as high as 72,000. If the population of centenarians continues to increase at its current rate of expansion, there could be close to 1 million people of 100 years of age or more by 2050 residing in the US. In the UK, while the overall number of centenarians is much smaller, the trend is the same. The Office of National Statistics reports around 9000 centenarians today in The UK and Wales, a 90-fold increase since 1911 and a 7% plus increase since 2005. At the current rate of expansion, the UK's centenarian population could reach over 40,000 by 2031. As in other parts of the industrialized world, people over 90 are the fastest growing segment of the population in the UK.

The East

In total numbers of centenarians, Japan is second to the US, with a current population of about 30,000, a number that has almost quadrupled in the last 10 years, meaning that the centenarian population in Japan has risen more dramatically then anywhere else. At its current rate of expansion, this age group in Japan may rival that of the United States in sheer numbers over the years ahead. Certainly, by 2050 Japan, proportionally, will have the most centenarians in the world. In proportion to its large population China does not have a high percentage of centenarians, about 7000 officially in the last census. With the rate of expansion of the population in general in China, and the number of centenarians increasing proportionally, it is estimated that in total numbers it will lead the world population of centenarians by 2050, with over 450,000.

Other Noteable Countries

The are many other places in the world having high numbers of centenarians, many of them claiming to have the "Most Centenarians" (in percentage terms) in the world. The most recent such claim goes to the Czech Republic where a just completed census shows that it has 673 centenarians in a population totaling approximately 10,500,000. Other countries with large centenarian populations include:

• Spain – 10,000

• France – Over 3000

• Canada – Circa 5000

• Italy – Circa 4750

Longevity, or at least extreme longevity, as in those who achieve the title of centenarian, does indeed seem to run in families. True there is the odd centenarian whose parents died young. It is also true that anyone can likely extend his or her lifespan by adopting the lifelong habits of centenarians. Regardless, researchers who study centenarians for clues on ageing constantly find the 100-year-old who "breaks all the rules". They have a poor diet, smoke, drink or like 104 year old Rhode Island native Michael Morowski, work in highly toxic environments. Michael was a coal miner for most for his life, but that did not stop him from becoming the oldest living person in

Rhode Island, recently taking part in the New England Centenarian Project.

Thomas Perls, director of the project found that Michael, like many other of the centenarians in the study, had a family history of longevity that stretched back at least two generations.

Quest for an Ageing Gene

Scientists have long sought a specific gene that determines lifespan. While no such "ageing gene" has yet to be found, there certainly seems to be a number of genetic factors that combine to influence who will live to 100. As in most things in the nature/nurture argument, seeing your 100th birthday seems to rely on a combination of both lifestyle and family history. The research seems to indicate that there is not a single gene that influences ageing, but in all of the centenarians studied, there appeared to be a number of common genetic traits that combined to help them age more slowly. Those few genes that were discovered that seemed to extend life, were mirrored for multiple generations. Clearly longevity runs in families and in some cases these genetic influences can be so strong that they overcome extremely toxic environments, as in the case of Mr. Morowski. Conversely, the study seemed to indicate that without at least some genetic basis to express long-life, it is unlikely that a person would reach extreme old age, , no matter how well they lived. That aside, a positive enviroment will allow any person to achieve the maximum lifespan his or her genes may predispose them to.

The Children of Centenarians

Current research also suggests that not only are children of centenarians more likely to reach 100 years of age themselves, they are far less likely to suffer from various life threatening illnesses, such as cardiovascular disease. The American Heart Association recently released the results of a study which concluded that grown children whose parents lived to be 100 years old or more, have a markedly lower incidence of heart disease, than those whose parents died in their 70s. The study also found that the children of centenarians had a lower risk factor of having a heart attack or stroke when they reached old age, than those whose parents died younger.

The research indicates that the children of centenarians have an advantage over the general population when it comes to cardiovascular health. In the study, researchers compared 176 children of centenarians with 166 controls. The adults in the control group had parents who were born in the same year as the centenarians, but who died in their mid-seventies. The average age of the offspring in the study was about the same, around 70 years of age, in both groups. When compared to the control group, the children of the centenarians had a 50% lower incidence of high blood pressure, heart disease, and diabetes.

It would seem that the genes of centenarians allow them to compress the time of greatest sickness and weakness into the very latest part of their lives. Almost invariably centenarians were relatively healthy through their 80's and into their 90's and only later did their health start to decline. Researchers concluded that if you have a strong family history for longevity, you probably have some genetic 'protection' and can afford to indulge a little bit in terms of lifestyle. But if you have a family history of heart disease, high blood pressure for example, you should do whatever you can now to put off what may otherwise be an inevitable illness in the later part of life.

There have been a number of centenarians that have accomplished amazing physical feats into their next century of life and most maintain at least some level of physical activity. According to centenarian researchers, a majority of the 100 year-old set does indeed maintain sharp minds and good cognitive function. The secret say the experts is to start now, and keep your brain functioning to its peak performance, long before you reach that triple digit birthday.

Preserving Cognitive abilities

Almost all of the centenarians interviewed by researchers said they keep up their mental faculties by engaging in stimulating mental activities that are both fun and interesting. Crossword puzzles are very popular among centenarians, as are card games and jigsaw puzzles, which can not only help keep the mind sharp, but when done with one or more partners, maintains a social interaction..

Anti-aging experts say that if you expect to live to 100, and want to enjoy it when you get there, the time to stretch your "brain muscles" is now. Challenge your mental capacity as much as possible. Take a stab at reading challenging books, complex technical or medical journals. Try learning one or more foreign languages, or take up a musical instrument.

Even learning a new dance can exercise your brain as well as your body. Believe it or not centenarians in Hawaii were taught, practiced, and performed the traditional hula dance. The intricacies of using the arm and hand movements to tell a story were a stimulating and mind-building exercise. Dance is an activity that requires coordination between multiple brain regions. So do many other artistic endeavours such as painting or drawing. These activities produce multiple benefits for the brain functions of centenarians.

A Simple Diet Plan for Longevity and Anti-Aging

The Longevity Diet Plan is a collection of practical eating guidelines that will help you be successful in changing your eating patterns in just one month. Eating healthier can become an obsession or sticking to a specific diet only makes eating more arduous and stressful than it should be. The trick to changing your eating habits for good is making a natural, simple change and this is the cornerstone of the longevity diet plan.

The way it works is this: you just follow one of the four healthy eating guidelines below each week to overhaul your diet and begin eating healthy without all the drama of a typical diet. The goal is to help you boost your healthy eating habits and curtail your bad eating habits one at a time. The focus is on what you can do better, instead of what you can't do food-wise. By focusing on the positive side of things, you make a better habit without putting too much attention into what you can't do.

Who Should Follow the Longevity Diet Plan?

Unlike most diets, the longevity plan is not a weight loss diet per se. Although the healthy habits that you start may lead to weight loss, the emphasis is on eating healthier. Do you want to eat healthier and make some changes to your diet, but don't want to follow a strict diet? The Longevity Diet is a month-long commitment, with a food challenge of sorts each week. The challenge calls for your eating real foods that are delicious as you make them to your liking. You'll need to invest some time in cooking and grocery shopping, but none in calorie counting. Here are the simple rules you follow on the longevity diet plan. As you follow along for a month or more, you'll become healthier every day.

The Rules of The Longevity Diet Plan

We give, then we take away. Each week, you'll make two changes to your diet. One change will involve adding something to your diet, the other change will involve removing or reducing something. It's the power of one, the simplicity of the challenge that will make it easy to follow along. After four weeks, you'll have eight simple rules about the foods you should and should not eat. That's all you'll need to remember – eight things:

• Double the Veggies, Hold the Cheese and the Milk (week one)

• Demote Meat and Go Nuts (week two)

• Get Fishy, No White Foods (week three)

• Love Fruit, Avoid Chemicals (week four)

The Results

You'll eat better, feel better and – although not designed as a weight loss plan – may even shed a few pounds. You will not have to think about complex food rules and make difficult decisions. The Longevity Diet is simple. Once you get the hang of the changes, you'll be able to easily increase your health through the foods you eat. So throw out those diet books and calorie charts and get started with the Longevity Diet today. You'll be happier, less stressed and healthier with this simple eating plan.

Avoid Smoking and Alcohol

People who do not smoke, are not obese, and consume alcohol moderately can expect to live seven years longer than the general population, and to spend most of these extra years in good health, according to a new study published today in Health Affairs.

People who refrain from engaging in risky health behaviours not only have a very long life -- longer than the famously long-lived Japanese -- but that most of these additional years of life are spent in good health.

The study, which analyzed data for more than 14,000 U.S. individuals, found that never-smokers who were not obese lived 4-5 years longer than the general population, and that these extra years were free of disability. The results of the analysis further indicated that individuals who also consumed alcohol moderately lived seven more disability-free years than the general population, and had a total life expectancy surpassing that of the population of Japan, a country that is often considered to be a vanguard of life expectancy. The study was conducted by Mikko Myrskylä, Director of the Max Planck Institute for Demographic Research, Germany; and Neil Mehta, Professor of Health Management and Policy at the University of Michigan, USA.

Several behaviours have a cumulative impact

"Improvements in medical technology are often thought to be the gatekeeper to healthier, longer life. We showed that a healthy lifestyle, which costs nothing, is enough to enable individuals to enjoy a very long and healthy life," said Mikko Myrskylä.

He added: "A moderately healthy lifestyle is enough to get the benefits. Avoiding becoming obese, not smoking, and consuming alcohol moderately is not an unrealistic goal."

This study was the first to analyze the cumulative impact of several key health behaviours on disability-free and total life expectancy. Previous studies have looked at single health behaviours. Mikko Myrskylä and his colleague instead examined several behaviors simultaneously, which allowed them to determine how long and healthy the lives of people who had avoided most of the well-known individual behavioral risk factors were.

Smoking and obesity affect health when aging

The researchers noted that each of the three unhealthy behaviours - obesity, smoking, and unhealthy consumption of alcohol - were linked to a reduction in life expectancy and to an earlier occurrence of disabilities.

But there were also differences: smoking was found to be associated with an early death but not with an increase in the number of years with disability, whereas obesity was shown to be associated with a long period of time with disability. Excessive alcohol consumption was found to be associated with both decreased lifespan and a reduced number of healthy years. However, the absence of all of these risky healthy behaviors was found to be associated with the greatest number of healthy years.

The most striking finding was the discovery of a large difference in average lifespan between the groups who were the most and the least at risk. Men who were not overweight, had never smoked, and drank moderately were found to live an average of 11 years longer than men who were overweight, had smoked, and drank excessively. For women, the gap between these two groups was found to be even greater, at 12 years.

"The most positive result is that the number of years that we have to live with physical limitations does not increase as we gain more years through healthy lifestyle. Instead, healthy lifestyle is associated with a strong increase in physically fit years. In other words, the years we gain through a healthy lifestyle are years in good health," said Mikko Myrskylä.

"Our results show how important it is to focus on prevention. Those who avoid risky health behaviours are achieving very long and healthy lives. Effective policy interventions targeting health behaviors could help larger fractions of the population to achieve the health benefits observed in this study," the researcher emphasized.

These results are important not only for individuals, but also for society. In an aging society, the health of the elderly determines the amount of money spent on the health system. In addition, healthy elderly people are better able to participate in the labor market and to perform social roles, such as caring for grandchildren.

The researchers used data from a long-term study conducted in the U.S., the Health and Retirement Study, which covered more than 14,000 individuals aged 50-89 over the 1998-2012 period. The participants were interviewed about their health and behaviors every two years. Those who reported having no limitations in the so-called activities of daily living (walking, dressing, bathing, getting out of bed, or eating) were classified as free of disability. The participants who had a body mass index of less than 30 were classified as not obese. Those who had smoked less than 100 cigarettes in their lifetime were considered never smokers. Men who had fewer than 14 drinks per week and women who had fewer than seven drinks per week were considered moderate drinkers. The researchers analyzed the ages at which the individuals with these healthy behaviours first became disabled, how many years they lived with disability, and their total life expectancy. The researchers then compared these results with those of the general population, and with those of individuals with particularly risky behavioural profiles.

According to the latest data collected by the National Center for Health statistics, poisoning, primarily by prescription drugs, has now surpassed car accidents as the leading cause of accidental death in the United States. In 2008, 41,000 Americans died from poisoning, compared to 38,000 lethal car accidents. The data, which can be found on the CDC's web siteiii, shows that:

• In 2008, poisoning became the leading cause of injury death in the United States and nearly 9 out of 10 poisoning deaths are caused by drugs.

• During the past three decades, the number of drug poisoning deaths increased six-fold from about 6,100 in 1980 to 36,500 in 2008.

• Opioid analgesics (prescription pain killers) were involved in more than 40 percent of all drug poisoning deaths in 2008, up from about 25 percent in 1999.

• During the most recent decade, the number of drug poisoning deaths involving opioid analgesics more than tripled from about 4,000 in 1999 to 14,800 in 2008.

While the drug poisoning death rate has risen among all age groups in the last decade, the death rate among adults between 45-54 is now the highest. Death by medicine is a 21st-century epidemic, and America's "war on drugs" is clearly directed at the wrong enemy when you consider that prescription drugs are now killing far more people than illegal drugs.

The most commonly abused prescription drugs like OxyContin, Vicodin, Xanax and Soma now cause more deaths than heroin and cocaine combined. In fact, prescription drugs are now the preferred "high" for many, especially teens, as they are typically used legally, which eliminates the stigma of being a "junkie."

Avoid Too Much of Fat and Sugar

You likely know that you should eat fat in moderation as excessive consumption of fat is bad for your health. Too much fat in your diet can cause a range of serious problems, including metabolic syndrome, cardiovascular disease and gastrointestinal issues. However, fat can also be a healthy part of your diet. Whether or not you're consuming too much fat comes down to the type of fat you're eating.

The health risks of eating too much fat are typically associated with the consumption of unhealthy fats. Fast foods, refined foods and processed foods, which are very popular in Western diets, are full of unhealthy fats.

According to a 2018 article in the American Journal of Lifestyle Medicine, at least 71 percent of Americans are overweight or obese. Many of these people suffer from other issues, like prediabetes or gastrointestinal inflammation.

Many of the dangers of eating too much fat start with minor issues — like weight gain, digestive problems, high blood pressure and high cholesterol. However, these problems can often be mediated by simply eating a healthier diet. In many cases, you don't even need to reduce your fat intake — you simply need to make sure you're consuming healthier fats.

Why Limiting Sugar is Key for Longevity

Limiting sugar in your diet is a well-known key to longevity, because of all the molecules capable of inflicting damage in your body, sugar molecules are probably the most damaging of all. Fructose in particular is an extremely potent pro-inflammatory agent that creates AGEs and speeds up the aging process. It also promotes the kind of dangerous growth of fat cells around your vital organs that are the hallmark of diabetes and heart disease. In one study on fructose, 16 volunteers on a controlled diet including high levels of fructose produced new fat cells around their heart, liver and other digestive organs in just 10 weeks!

Sugar/fructose also increases your insulin and leptin levels and decreases receptor sensitivity for both of these vital hormones, and this is another major factor of premature aging and age-related chronic degenerative diseases such as heart disease. Keep in mind that while it's perfectly normal for your blood sugar levels to rise slightly after every meal, it is not natural or healthy when your blood sugar levels become excessively elevated and stay that way.

Unfortunately, that's exactly what will happen if you're eating like the stereotypical American, who consumes a staggering 2.5 pounds of sugar a week on average!

And when you add in other low-quality carb foods such as white bread, sugar, pasta, pastries, cookies, and candy, which also break down to sugar in your body, it's not so difficult to see why so many Americans are in such poor health.

This type of high-sugar (high-carb) diet is also what's driving the obesity epidemic—notdiets high in fat. An infographic created by Column Five for Massive Health, based on Why We Get Fat by science writer Gary Taubes, explains why. In short, carbs, like fructose and other sugars, destroy your insulin and leptin sensitivity, which in turn causes your cells to accumulate more fat, and makes it more difficult to get rid of the extra weight as well. So, the bottom line is this: If you want to look and feel younger longer, avoid all forms of sugar (including grains) as much as possible!

The Anti-Aging Lifestyle

Of all the healthy lifestyle strategies I know of that can have a significant impact on your longevity, normalizing your insulin and leptin levels is probably the most important. Cutting out sugar and grains and increasing exercise are two effective ways to accomplish that.

But to truly optimize your longevity and slow down the clock, your entire lifestyle needs to be taken into account. So, here are the rest of my top "anti-aging" recommendations. Incorporating these healthy lifestyle guidelines will help set you squarely on the path to optimal health and give you the best shot at living a much longer life:

• Learn how to effectively cope with stress – Stress has a direct impact on inflammation, which in turn underlies many of the chronic diseases that kill people prematurely every day, so developing effective coping mechanisms is a major longevity-promoting factor.

Meditation, prayer, physical activity and exercise are all viable options that can help you maintain emotional and mental equilibrium. I also strongly believe in using energy psychology tools such as the Emotional Freedom Technique (EFT) to address deeper, oftentimes hidden emotional problems.

• Eat a healthy diet focused on whole, ideally organic, foods – My nutrition plan, based on natural whole foods, is your first step toward increasing your chances of living a longer, healthier life.

• Optimize Your Vitamin D Levels. This is another very powerful and inexpensive intervention that can have profound benefits on your health. In the summer you can do this for free by careful and safe sun exposure. In the winter a therapeutic level of oral vitamin D can be achieved with an oral supplement (around 8,000 units of vitamin D3 a day for most adults)

• Animal based omega-3 fats – Correcting the ratio of omega-3 to healthful omega-6 fats is a strong factor in helping you live longer. This typically means increasing your intake of animal based omega-3 fats, such as krill oil, while decreasing your intake of damaged omega-6 fats (think trans fats).

I do not, however, recommend the new prescription strength fish oil medication, sold under the name Lovaza. Don't be fooled by their "all-natural" PR campaign. This is actually a drug to treat very high triglyceride levels. However, as with most other drugs, Lovaza comes with potentially dangerous side effects that you would not experience with a natural fish oil or krill oil supplement. Side effects include flu-like symptoms, infections, back pain, skin rashes, upset stomach, taste changes, digestive issues, chest pain, migraines and respiratory problems!

Additionally, new research strongly suggests that 500 mg of krill oil is more potent and far less expensive.

• Get your antioxidants from foods –Good sources include blueberries, cranberries, blackberries, raspberries, strawberries, cherries, beans, and artichokes.

• Use coconut oil – Another excellent anti-aging food is coconut oil, known to reduce your risk of heart disease and lower your cholesterol, among other things. In fact, it's doubly beneficial because it can be both eaten and applied directly to your skin. Coconut oil can be used in place of other oils, margarine, butter, or shortening, and can be used for all your cooking needs.

• Get your resveratrol naturally – Resveratrol is one of the forerunners in the anti-aging pill race, but more than likely, by the time they've manipulated it into a synthetic pill (like the fish oil discussed above), it won't be healthy for you.

Although resveratrol is the antioxidant found in red wine, I can't recommend drinking wine in the hopes of extending your life because alcohol is a neuro toxin that can poison your brain and harm your body's delicate hormonal balance. Instead, get your resveratrol from natural sources, such as whole grape skins and seeds, raspberries, mulberries, and peanuts.

• Exercise regularly and smartly - Studies repeatedly show that regular, moderate-to-vigorous exercise can help prevent or delay your onset of hypertension, obesity, heart disease, osteoporosis, and the falls that lead to hip fracture. Although a lifetime of regular exercise is ideal, it's never too late to start. It has been shown that even individuals in their 70's can substantially increase both strength and endurance with exercise.

High-intensity, interval training can also increase longevity as this specific style of training promotes human growth hormone production – yet another aspect of the longevity puzzle.

• Avoid as many chemicals, toxins, and pollutants as possible – This includes tossing out your toxic household cleaners, soaps, personal hygiene products, air fresheners, bug sprays, lawn pesticides, and insecticides, just to name a few, and replacing them with non-toxic alternatives.

• Avoid pharmaceutical drugs – Pharmaceutical drugs kill thousands of people prematurely every year – as an expected side effect of the action of the drug. And, if you adhere to a healthy lifestyle, you most likely will never need any of them in the first place.

Sports and Exercise

Being active is good for you on so many levels, from keeping the heart in shape to improving blood pressure and blood sugar levels. Exercise has also been linked to benefits for the brain and lower risk of some cancers.

But which types of activity pack the best health punch? Does it matter what kind of exercise you do?

In a study published in the British Journal of Sports Medicine, European and Australian researchers find that not all types of physical activity are equal when it comes to longevity. They studied data collected from more than 80,000 people in England and Scotland who answered questions about their activity levels yearly between 1994 and 2008. The data showed that people who engaged in three types of exercise—racquet sports like tennis or racquet ball, swimming and aerobics—had the lowest risk of dying during the study period.

Overall, 44% of the people met recommended public health exercise levels. (That's 150 minutes of moderate-to-vigorous activity each week in the U.S.) Among those that did, people who played racquet sports had a 47% lower risk of dying during the nine-year study than people who didn't exercise. Swimmers had a 28% lower risk of death and those doing aerobics showed a 27% lower risk of dying. These were the reductions after the scientists adjusted for factors that might affect early death, like smoking.

Runners surprisingly did not show a lower risk of mortality during the study, but lead study author Pekka Oja, retired scientific director for the UKK Institute for Health Promotion Research in Finland, says that may be explained by the fact that most of the runners were younger than those engaging in the other sports. They may need to be followed for a longer period of time to assess their death rates.

Cycling also was associated with a relatively smaller drop in mortality risk, possibly because many of the people who reported cycling did it recreationally or to get to and from work and were less likely to work up a sweat and have a vigorous workout. Swimming and racquet sports, on the other hand, inherently require a pretty intense level of exercise.

That's why Oja says people shouldn't interpret the results as endorsing one type of activity over another. The bottom line: people who exercised had lower mortality overall than people who didn't. "They are all good," he says of all types of physical activity. "It's up to individuals to decide what they like and their circumstances for participating in different activities."

Much scientific research has shown that dogs have a positive impact on a human's life, physically and psychologically. If you are a dog parent, I suppose we don't need to talk about how your dog makes you happy any further. But, did you know that owning a dog makes your social life better too?

There are roughly 4 million dogs in the United States, which means there are at least 3,999,999 people out there that can connect with you through a topic about dogs. It is natural to ask a random stranger about which park they take their dogs to, which is the best dry dog food for Pitbulls, in their opinion, or to share a cute moment, as long as a dog is by their side.

Dogs need exercise, so dog owners tend to have a greater requirement for daily activities than other people. Not only your walk, hike or run will be more interesting, but your relationship with your dog will be deepened. It will open new opportunities to talk to others on your hiking trails or while in dog parks. Starting and maintaining new friendships is easier with the positive vibes coming from your dog.

By taking care of a dog, owners can add more structure and routine to their day. Stress often makes us depressed and anxious, but faced with a simple plaintive look from a pup will make you want to get out of bed and join him in exercising. With a consistent routine, humans tend to be more balanced and calm, and symptoms of depression, bipolar disorder, and PTSD are reduced.

People with emotional difficulties can find a lot of help in dogs. Dogs and cats have therapeutic effects, as they fulfill our needs for touch. One study found out that hardened criminals show long-term changes in their behavior after frequent exposure to dogs. Many of them say that interacting with a dog helped them feel mutual affection for the first time in their life. By the touch of a canine, our sensory stress is relieved, making our mind more open.

Isolation and loneliness often trigger for depression. Caring for a living animal makes people feel needed and wanted, distract them from their own problems, and reduce their risk of depression by to 34%. The loyal and warm companionship of a dog is proven to prevent illness and increase longevity.

If you are struggling with social life or emotional problems, you might consider adopting a dog to help with these problems. The presence of a dog will offer you comfort, help you build self-confidence, reduce anxiety and open the chances to make new friends. That's how owning a dog makes your social life better.

Eat Quality Food Instead of Industrial Food

Food and what it can do for us has become a question of concern. We all think of food as a life-giving resource, but it's interesting to know that the same food that we think is giving us life can also be damaging to us.

In a modern diet, we eat many foods that are not good for us. Because of the ease of preparing processed foods, we are eating a lot of unhealthy fats and by doing this we are actually causing a lot of our own health problems. Food can be directly linked to many different diseases. Therefore, it's essential that we watch what we eat and how we eat it.

Knowing the effects of food and changing our habits are two completely different things. If we could pursue a healthier and happier existence by resetting our taste for food and taking on different habits, why don't we?

The answer is a combination of factors. One reason is that we have become addicted to our modern diet that is high in sugar and salt, both of which can be very addictive. Our taste buds have gotten accustomed to high levels of sugar and salt, and so when we eat natural foods, we find them bland. But if you were to spend some time away from processed foods and take the time to get used to fresh fruits and vegetables, your taste buds will get accustomed to the subtle but satisfying taste of natural foods. Another reason is that a lot of well-meaning doctors and nutrition experts end up giving advice that is counterproductive and causes more harm than help.

If we go back fifty years or so, medical conditions such as obesity, diabetes, arthritis and food allergies were relatively rare, but have now become commonplace. The reason is our our modern Western diet, not only are people fatter, but they are also sicker than ever before.

Everywhere modern processed goods go, chronic disease including obesity, diabetes, and heart disease goes as well. Although there are a number of factors that contribute to these chronic health problems, our diet is the most important.

Over the past 160 years, our total sugar intake has skyrocketed. People in Western-diet countries are consuming about 150 pounds of sugar a year, which is over 500 calories a day of sugar!

Added sugar is a contributor to not only obesity, but also diabetes, heart disease, and cancer because sugar promotes inflammation. Worse yet is the consumption of soda and fruit juice. One study found that in children, sugar-sweetened beverages are responsible for a 60 percent increase in obesity.

People have abandoned traditional fats in favor of highly processed or hydrogenated vegetable oils. I just read a statement by a cardiologist telling people to replace butter with a canola oil spread. When health professionals blame saturated fats for heart disease, people will abandon them in favor of processed oils. However, these oils are high in omega-6 fats, which contribute to inflammation. Therefore, the misguided advice to avoid saturated fats and replace them with highly processed vegetable oils might actually be responsible for the heart disease epidemic that we see today.

Egg consumption has also decreased because of misguided advice. Eggs are one of the most nutritious foods. Although eggs are high in cholesterol, there is no evidence that they raise bad cholesterol or contribute to heart disease. As a result of this misguided advice, we have substituted refined, highly processed, and sugared boxed cereals for eggs.

Since 1950, we have decreased our egg consumption by 33 percent, while heart disease has skyrocketed. Not only this, but people are eating more processed foods than ever before.

Elements of a Traditional Diet

In a traditional diet, food comes from the source. This means that the fruits and vegetables come from the ground, meat comes from the animal, and bread and other goods come from baking from scratch. Nothing comes from a factory, nothing is processed.

By taking the time to ensure that we know that our food is free from chemicals and hormones, we ensure that we are putting natural elements into our bodies rather than trusting a box to tell us that the contents are healthy. Based on how "morally" other big corporations have behaved in the past, can we really trust our health to food corporations?

A hundred years ago, people ate a traditional diet because that was all there was. Everything was organic.

Nowadays, we are seeing people die younger due to heart disease and other factors that can be directly linked to our diet. Obviously, the people who enjoyed longevity a century ago had the right idea as to what and when they ate.

According to a Weston A. Price Foundation article "Modernizing Your Diet with Traditional Foods," by Joette Calabrese, all traditional cultures:

* Consume some sort of animal protein, including organ meats and fat, every day

* Consume foods that contain very high levels of minerals and fat-soluble vitamins (vitamin A, vitamin D, and vitamin K2 found in seafood, organ meats, and animal fats)

* Consume some foods with high enzyme and probiotic content

* Consume seeds, grains, and nuts that are soaked, sprouted, fermented, or naturally leavened in order to neutralize a portion of the naturally occurring anti-nutrients in these foods

* Consume plenty of natural fats, but no industrial liquid or hardened (partially hydrogenated) oils

* Consume natural, unrefined salt

* Consume animal bones, usually in the form of gelatin-rich bone broths

* Provide extra nutrition for parents-to-be, pregnant women, breastfeeding women, and growing children, to ensure the health of the next generation

* Do not consume refined or processed foods, including white flour, refined sweeteners, pasteurized and low-fat milk products, protein powders, industrial fats and oils, and chemical additives

These are suggestions to work toward because simple, time-proven foods can make a huge difference in your health and longevity.

Although every person has unique food preferences and needs, studies have proven that the traditional diet consistently promotes longevity and vitality.

The traditional diet is time proven. There are many people all over the world who have been eating the same way for thousands of years—look at India, Mexico, and China for proof. These people are living longer, healthier lives even today. Knowing that people are living longer due to their diets is key to understanding the message of this chapter. If you were to ask centenarians what their secret to longevity is, they would name what they eat as one of the main factors. People who eat better live longer.

I want to encourage you to think before you shop and before you eat. Now that you see that food has a direct impact upon your health, try to make the necessary changes in your diet to ensure that you don't meet a premature death due to poor eating, or a compromised old age spent hobbling between infirmaries. I encourage all who read this to try to take on a more traditional diet. Your body will thank you!

Although we can't all eat the way those people eat, here are some changes you can make right now:

* Wherever possible shop at local farmer's markets

* Buy hormone-free eggs and wild fish instead of farmed

* Buy grass-fed meats and dairy products

* Purchase foods that do not come in a package

* Try to use more natural sweeteners instead of refined sugar

* Choose whole grains instead of white flour

* Cook at home—home cooking is best; cooking with fire rather than a microwave   is better

* Include seasonal and locally grown fruits and vegetables in your diet

* Include legumes, beans, nuts, and seeds

* Buy seasonal foods

Long-Term Health or Transient Gratification?

Taking responsibility for our health means a commitment to change. We must be prepared to abandon lifelong habits. Most of us love our indulgences, and giving them up seems a terrible deprivation, but we cannot restore our health until we begin to place a higher value on our health than on the immediate and transient gratification that we get from certain foods.

Health is not merely the absence of disease, but it is also a state of optimum well-being from which life seems to flow effortlessly. When the body is healthy, the mind is healthy and our judgment is on target. We seem to always be "in the right place at the right time." Our intuition becomes strong and enables us to function harmoniously within our environment. The way we eat can help us enjoy life with greater health and vitality.

Eat Less Meat

Americans who ate a diet rich in animal protein during middle age were significantly more likely to die from cancer and other causes, compared with people who reported going easy on foods such as red meat and cheese, fresh research suggests.

The study, published Tuesday in the journal Cell Metabolism, was based on an analysis of data from NHANES, an ongoing federally funded study that surveys Americans about their eating habits and behaviors.

In this particular study, researchers tracked about 6,000 older adults included in the survey to find connections between dietary patterns, death and disease.

"The research shows that a low-protein diet in middle age is useful for preventing cancer and overall mortality," wrote co-author Eileen Crimmins, the AARP Chair in Gerontology at the University of Southern California, in a release about the paper.

But here's the catch: The researchers also found that for older people, ages 65 and up, there may be a benefit to eating more protein. In this age group, higher levels of protein seemed to be protective against cancer and premature death.

So how might these age-dependent effects be explained? Well, Valter Longo, the director of the Longevity Institute at USC, who led the research, points to changes in the growth hormone known as IGF-I.

When we're young, IGF-1 help promotes growth, which is good. But as we age, too much protein in our diets may lead to overly high levels of IGF-1, which may contribute to aging and DNA damage, Longo explains.

Then, after 65, when IGF-I levels trail off, our bodies may benefit from more protein in the diet to help fend of frailty and decline.

"We've suspected that this is the case," Longo tells The Salt. In his view, most middle-aged Americans are eating too much protein.

The findings, he says, build on previous research he's done on IGF-I, including a studythat looked at a group of Ecuadorians who had low levels of cancer and diabetes due to a genetic mutation that lowered levels of IGF-I.

In the new study, Longo and his colleagues found that high-protein foods derived from plants, such as beans and nuts, did not have the same effect on mortality as did high-protein foods from animals.

Singling out the effects of protein in the diet is hard to do. For starters, our diets are complex, and sussing out the independent effect of any one component is tough. What's more, surveying people on what they have eaten, as NHANES does, and then trying to figure out how that influences their health years later is a tricky business. So there are still lots of questions about how to interpret these findings.

In an age when advocates of the Paleo Diet and other low-carb eating plans such as Atkins talk up the virtues of protein because of its satiating effects, expect plenty of people to be skeptical of the new findings.

That said, as we've previously reported, several other studies have found a link between a high intake of red meat — especially processed meats like bacon and salami — and other animal proteins and an increased risk of mortality.

But could eating meat and cheese really be as bad for you as smoking, as the university news release describing the new Cell Metabolism paper suggested?

Well, that may be an exaggeration, according to Dr. Frank Hu, a researcher at the Harvard School of Public Health who studies the links between health, diet and lifestyle.

"The harmful effects of smoking on cancer and mortality are well-established to be substantial, while the harmful effects of red meat consumption are modest in comparison," Hu wrote to us in an email.

For instance, in a study Hu authored, people who ate a serving of red meat every day had a 13 percent increased risk of mortality, compared with those who ate little meat. By comparison, people who swapped out red meat for alternative sources of protein cut their risk of premature death. Choosing chicken and other poultry decreased the risk by 14 percent, fish decreased the risk by 7 percent and legumes decreased the risk by 10 percent.

So the debate about how much protein is ideal — and from which sources — will go on. In the meantime, if you're feeling confused, consider the one strategy that almost all experts agree on: moderation. The simplest way to maintain a healthy body weight and cut the risk of so many weight-related diseases is to limit calories.

So eat what you enjoy. Upsize servings of greens and other vegetables. And downsize servings of meat, cheese and other high-calorie foods.

In addition, eating less meat is better for the planet. Meat consumption and livestock are the largest source of CO_2 emissions on earth, ahead of transport. A reduction in the proportion of meat in the diet could stem the phenomenon of global warming.

Fasting To Detoxify

Fasting is currently one of, if not the, most popular eating pattern these days and is believed to be an important therapeutic tool for longevity.

Well-nourished calorie restriction (fasting) can enhance healthy aging in a number of ways. Perhaps most easily observable to the naked eye are reductions in waist circumference and total body fat while preserving lean body mass – all improvements in metabolic syndrome conditions. Metabolic syndrome is a cluster of conditions that includes high blood pressure, high blood sugar, excess abdominal fat, and high cholesterol and triglycerides which increase a person's risk for heart disease, stroke, and diabetes – all common preventable diseases.

Beyond healthy weight reduction, even more is taking place at a cellular level while fasting. Insulin-like growth factor 1 (IGF-1), mammalian target of rapamycin (mTOR), and protein kinase A (PKA) are three nutrient pathways associated with age-related disease, specifically longevity, cellular growth, and metabolism, respectively. Done effectively, fasting has been shown to improve outcomes with each of these three important markers of metabolic health as well as promoting improvement in C-Reactive Protein (CRP), a nonspecific metabolic marker of inflammation.

Fasting has a positive impact on lipids as triglycerides, cholesterol, HDL, and LDL values all show improvements when fasting. The CALERIE2 trial in 2015 in which calories were simply restricted by 25% over a 2-year period showed improvements in insulin resistance, cholesterol, and blood pressure while revealing no untoward effects on quality of life of participants. This makes sense since we know cholesterol synthesis occurs in a fed state and cholesterol breakdown occurs in an unfed, or fasting, state where it can be utilized for cellular repair and energy.

This begs the question – why isn't fasting recommended more often for lipid management instead of statins?

Cellular regeneration and detoxification, DNA repair, mitochondrial health, and cell recycling are additional benefits of fasting as cleansing and regeneration are a part of cholesterol breakdown. As our cells detoxify, we also reduce our inflammatory pathways, which can translate to reduction of joint and body pain. Autophagy is the process of recycling our body's own damaged tissues into useable energy when we fast.

Further, when our body begins this process of autophagy, stem cell production is stimulated which ought to capture everyone's attention these days. Stem cells are undifferentiated cells with the ability to grow into any of the body's 200 types of cells, thus truly promoting regeneration, healing and anti-aging.

As stated above, there are several indicators pointing towards fasting as an effective approach to health management and longevity when done healthfully. Intermittent fasting (IF), periodic fasting (PF) and fast-mimicking (FM) are each a different approach to fasting, and I recommend you discuss the nuances between them with your doctor or qualified health practitioner who can help navigate you towards optimal health and wellness.

Avoid Stress

Reducing stress in your everyday life is vital for maintaining your overall health, as it can improve your mood, boost immune function, promote longevity and allow you to be more productive. When you let your stress get the best of you, you put yourself at risk of developing a range of illnesses – from the common cold to severe heart disease. Stress has such a powerful impact on your well being because it is a natural response that is activated in the brain. Let's examine how this process works, why stress affects you the way it does, and the severe impacts it can have on your health.

The Science of Stress

When you become stressed, the brain undergoes both chemical and physical changes that affect its overall functioning. During periods of high stress, certain chemicals within the brain, including the neurotransmitters dopamine, epinephrine and norepinephrine begin to rise, causing larger amounts of these and other "fight-or-flight" hormones such as adrenalin to be released by the adrenal glands. The release of these chemicals contributes to certain physiological effects, including rapid heart rate, higher blood pressure, and a weakened immune system. When left unmanaged over time, chronic stress can lead to the development of other serious problems, such as stomach ulcers, stroke, asthma, and heart disease.

Sleep Well at Night

A good night's sleep could be the key to better health and even to living longer.

There has been mounting evidence that sleep may hold a key for health and well-being, but recent studies indicate that it may also play a role in how long you live.

Sleep deprivation has been linked to health problems such as obesity, negative mood and behavior, decreased productivity, and safety issues in the home, on the job and on the road. Fragmented or insufficient sleep also raises levels of blood fats, cholesterol, cortisol and blood pressure – all powerful risk factors for heart disease.

Not getting enough sleep each night – or even getting too much sleep – may also increase your risk of developing type 2 diabetes, according to research conducted at Yale University. It was reported that men getting no more than six hours of sleep per night, as well as those getting more than eight hours, were at significantly increased risk for developing diabetes, compared to men getting seven to eight hours of sleep each night. Habitual sleep restriction could play a very important role in increasing risk for diabetes later in life, especially if maintained over many years and decades.

Now, recent studies have looked at the link between sleep and longevity. One study, published recently in the Sleep journal, found that people who get less than six hours sleep per night have an increased risk of dying prematurely; those who slumbered for less than that amount of time were 12 percent more likely to die early. Researchers also found a link between sleeping more than nine hours and premature death, but said oversleeping is more likely to be an effect of illness, rather than a cause.

Another study found that people who reach 100 are three times more likely to spend at least 10 hours a night in bed. Those over the age of 100 reporting they have a good night's rest were 70 percent higher than participants younger than 79 years of age. In this study, people who said they were in bad health were more likely to have poor sleeping patterns.

Sleep experts say most adults, regardless of age, need between seven and nine hours a sleep each night for optimum performance, health and safety.

But as we get older, we tend to sleep less, and there is increased fragmentation of sleep; older people wake up more often and for longer periods of time during the night. For older people with health problems, their condition can have an impact on their sleep.

And most age-related diseases will affect sleep and will be affected by sleep (or the lack of it). For example, painful conditions like arthritis or back pain will affect sleep by causing arousal during the night. Sleep-related breathing disorders, which tend to be more frequent in older individuals, may affect quality of sleep and cause sleep deprivation, resulting in additional health problems.

So how do we get enough of the restorative, replenishing sleep that we need? There are lifestyle steps you can take before you go to bed that can help you fall asleep and get better sleep. Read Dr. Cherry's Guidelines for Better Sleep for his tips. You can also listen to or read the summary from Dr. Cherry's May 6 radio program, in which he talks about natural ways to enhance your quality of sleep.

His natural approach includes Sleep Support, a combination of nine natural herbs, vitamins, minerals and extracts in one safe, effective, non-habit-forming formulation. It may be just what you need for a peaceful night's rest – and optimal health.

Not Working Too Hard After Certain Age

It's long been said that always looking at the positive side of things and not working too hard will lead to a long and happy life, but a new study by University of California, Riverside researchers has challenged those beliefs.

"It's surprising just how often common assumptions - by both scientists and the media - are wrong," said Howard S. Friedman, distinguished professor of psychology who led the 20-year study.

Friedman and Leslie R. Martin, a 1996 UCR alumna (Ph.D.) and staff researchers, examined, refined and supplemented data gathered by the late Stanford University psychologist Louis Terman and subsequent researchers on more than 1,500 bright children who were about 10 years old when they were first studied in 1921.

"Probably our most amazing finding was that personality characteristics and social relations from childhood can predict one's risk of dying decades later," Friedman concluded.

The study followed the children through their lives, collecting information that included family histories and relationships, teacher and parent ratings of personality, hobbies, pet ownership, job success, education levels, military service and numerous other details.

"When we started, we were frustrated with the state of research about individual differences, stress, health and longevity," Friedman recalled. "It was clear that some people were more prone to disease, took longer to recover, or died sooner, while others of the same age were able to thrive. All sorts of explanations were being proposed - anxiety, lack of exercise, nerve-racking careers, risk-taking, lack of religion, unsociability, disintegrating social groups, pessimism, poor access to medical care, and Type A behavior patterns."

But none were well-studied over the long term. That is, none followed people step-by-step throughout their lives.

When Friedman and Martin began their research in 1991, they planned to spend six months examining predictors of health and longevity among the Terman participants.

But the project continued over the next two decades and the team eventually involved more than 100 graduate and undergraduate students who tracked down death certificates, evaluated interviews, and analyzed tens of thousands of pages of information about the Terman participants through the years.

"We came to a new understanding about happiness and health," said Martin, now a psychology professor at La Sierra University in Riverside. "One of the findings that really astounds people, including us, is that the Longevity Project participants who were the most cheerful and had the best sense of humor as kids lived shorter lives, on average, than those who were less cheerful and joking. It was the most prudent and persistent individuals who stayed healthiest and lived the longest."

The study also found that "don't work too hard, don't stress" doesn't work as advice for good health and long life. Terman subjects who were the most involved and committed to their jobs did the best.

Drink Coffe and Organic Tee

Drinking a cup of roasted organic coffee in the morning may be one of the best things you can do all day to stay healthy and live a long life. Over the years, researchers have found overwhelming evidence about coffee's health benefits. But now, scientists are really beginning to understand the causal mechanisms that help explain just how coffee helps keeps aging and disease at bay.

Why coffee is an antioxidant powerhouse

You can think of coffee as a plant-based medicine. It is packed with phytonutrients, antioxidants and (of course) caffeine. When most people think of antioxidant foods they think of berries, artichokes and spices like turmeric. But medium roast Arabica coffee has an oxygen radical absorbance capacity (ORAC) score of 2,780. That means coffee is a more potent free radical scavenger than good sources like pomegranate juice, broccoli, cardamon spices, green tea, organic red wine and apples.

The fact that coffee can more than hold its own against fruits and vegetables as a source of antioxidants will surprise lots of people. Another unexpected revelation is how beneficial caffeine can be. Plants developed this compound as a defense mechanism (to ward off predatory insects). But scientists have discovered that caffeine, in addition to being a natural stimulant, has both powerful antioxidant and anti-inflammatory properties.

Scientists believe that coffee's formidable capacity to counteract inflammation is key to its ability to both prevent and reverse disease. Recently, for instance, researchers at the Institute for Immunity, Transplantation and Infection at Stanford University in California discovered clear evidence that caffeine targets gene clusters that produce inflammation linked to cardiovascular disease. The results of their study, which were published in the journal Nature Medicine, strongly suggest that drinking three to five cups of coffee a day effectively shortcircuits inflammatory processes that are associated with heart disease, hypertension and strokes.

Do Not Take Dietary Supplements

If you've gone to a dietician, you've probably been warned against diet supplements. and you probably already know that they can contain both healthy and unhealthy ingredients. That means there are tons of unhealthy ingredients in diet supplements to avoid — if you value your health.

Healthy diet supplements often involve boosts of protein, green tea, and vitamins. In other words, these supplements are often found in food and are made to help encourage overall health and wellness rather than weight loss in most cases.

Unhealthy ingredients in diet supplements are way more common, and they're often focused on weight loss. In some cases, they're just bad for your wallet and give you the jitters. In other cases, they can end up with a trip to the hospital - or even the morgue.

You might wonder how unhealthy or fraudulent diet supplements even make it onto the market. After all, the FDA was made to test out medicines and food, and they wouldn't just turn a blind eye to this stuff, right?

Well, not quite. The fact is that diet supplements aren't regulated by the Food and Drug Administration. This is why many dangerous dietary supplements are often used - and why no one actually seems to notice.

So, if you take diet pills or other similar dietary supplements, read the ingredients and make sure your supplementation is healthy!

Lead A Balanced and Healthy Life

Living a healthy lifestyle may mean something different from one person to the next. For some, health is defined by living a disease-free life. For others, healthy is being able to play with grandchildren or perhaps adhering to a weekly exercise schedule. Though the definition of healthy may differ between people, living a healthy lifestyle is a fundamental component to achieving your optimal mental and physical well-being.

According to the authors of a March 2003 study published in "Age and Ageing," people who engage in unhealthy habits -- such as smoking, a poor quality diet, and physical inactivity, are at increased risk for premature health decline and death. Though many factors contribute to your overall health, diet and physical activity are leading determinants of your level of health and quality of life. A nutritious diet of whole grains, lean meats, vegetables, fruits and healthy fats is necessary for weight management. A balanced diet also helps maintain energy levels throughout the day. Regular physical activity, which includes a variety of aerobic and strength-building exercises, prevents weight gain that can lead to a plethora of chronic conditions. Additionally, lifestyle habits -- such as not smoking and limiting alcohol intake -- contribute to a healthy life. Allowing your body to rest each day by getting a proper amount of sleep is also important to achieving a healthy lifestyle.

The Power of Plants

One final subject for you to consider. Children more concentrated at school, patients who recover from ill health faster, employees more motivated: the panacea is on our doorstep. And to believe the researchers, it only takes one thing to make life sweeter: plants.

For more than 30 years, researchers have been interested in the beneficial effects of plants on human health. Fifteen minutes in a forest, and participants in a Japanese study felt less anxious, less angry and more vigorous, effects that a walk in town would not bring unfortunately.

Even those who find themselves in hospital are better off when their rooms overlook a natural landscape. In 1984, an American study showed that patients undergoing gallbladder surgery were less likely to have complications, consumed fewer painkillers, and left the hospital earlier when they simply had a view of trees.

"Nature has an analgesic side and provides well-being, which even influences the healing time," says Stefan Jordy, researcher at the University of South Brittany and member of the only French team specialized on the issue.

Nature also boosts the immune system. Not only will a walk in the forest make you happier, it will also allow the body to produce more killer cells, those lymphocytes that are at the forefront of human immunity. Virtues that other cultures are not unaware of: in Japanese medicine, "shinrin-yoku" is to send the sick cures in the forest, to treat the most diverse diseases.

According to research, the benefits of nature will be exactly the same whether it's a hike, a tree view, a green plant on the shelf, or even a photographic image. We therefore know that it is through the gaze that nature has its benefits and not through a chemical substance. Put simply, nature meets an archaic need of human beings. The reason for this is that nature confirms to us that one of our absolute requirements for survival, water, is present. We become less stressed on a deep sub-conscious level because that basic need has been fulfilled. This is a similar response to those animals in a zoo which are happier when that are better off when their surroundings look like their natural habitat.

For others, more inspired by poetry, it is thanks to its beauty that nature allows us to relax our attention for a moment, and to recharge our batteries, in a way. In one classroom, for example, a study showed that students learn best when plants decorate the room. Results that have been replicated in the corporate environment: employees are more satisfied with their working conditions, are absent less often and work better as a team when plants decorate offices.

Not content to make people happy, nature also creates social bonds. In one experiment, a researcher dropped an object "inadvertently" and observed the number of people who helped to pick it up. Depending on where the experiment was conducted, either in a natural landscape or in an urban environment, the proportion of good Samaritans increased from 50% to 80%. We can only conclude that people are more inclined to help each other when surrounded by nature than in the city when we display more self-centered tendencies.

Many urban planners have recognized the beneficial effect of greenery and in France, for instance, urban planners, architects and decision-makers now take this into consideration when building new developments to enhance the surroundings of those that will live there. Back in Brittany, Jordy and his colleagues have been assisting a local health clinic by putting plants throughout the building to the benefit of its patients, claiming it to be a "win-win approach" with healthier patients and the costs saved through their quicker recovery. All this, for the price of some plants.

Conclusion

Currently, there are more people over the age of 65 than at any time in history. There are many theories as to why some people tend to live longer these days, but no doubt genetics plays a huge role. However, the latest studies indicate that of those who live into their 90s and 100s, only 35 percent have the longevity gene. Len Kravitz (2015), professor of exercise science at the University of New Mexico, spoke on the dynamics of longevity and said that we need to adapt a philosophy of "healthspan" instead of "lifespan."

Kravitz says that in order to maintain optimal healthspan, the following are essential: minimizing stress, maintaining physical activity, keeping your brain active, socializing, and laughing more.

In order to create or maintain a healthy lifestyle well into one's golden years, Kravitz also suggests shedding pounds, if necessary. Being overweight as a result of a poor diet is a major contributor to declining health and well-being as we age. According to the Centers for Disease Control and Prevention (CDC), close to 80 million adults in the U.S. are obese. Obesity-related conditions include heart disease, stroke, type 2 diabetes, and certain types of cancer.

"Chronic stress is also a big contributor to aging," Kravitz said, "and the best way to fight it is with exercise. Incorporate some resistance training, aerobic exercise and mind/body practices to deal with stress at work or wherever the problem exists. When you take this multi-faceted approach, you can mediate the stress and have less cognitive decline as well."

Pietri et al. (2017) studied the island of Ikaria, a small island in the Aegean Sea that has one of the world's longest-living populations. Apparently, centenarians were on the island as many as 400 years ago. Pietri correlated the increased chance of longevity there to factors such as air, water, community spirit, sparse diet, and inherited disposition. In essence, these people live on one of the very poorest islands, yet they are the happiest and live the longest of all those in the entire Aegean Sea.

Food for thought indeed.

About the author

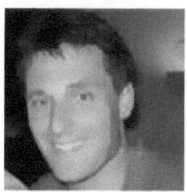

Nicolas Huvet was born in 1972, the product of a French father and a Swedish mother and as such his childhood was influenced greatly by the culture of both countries.

Following attaining his scientific bachelor's degree in 1990, he went on to the University of Paris Villetaneuse, where he obtained a Bachelor of Science (mathematics option) in 1993. This was followed by military service in the air force, after which he pursued two years of additional studies to obtain a master of logistics transport.

His working life began in the field of air and sea transport in which he worked tirelessly between 1997 and 2007, also obtaining a master's degree of logistics during this time.

He then went to work in Stockholm, for a computer science company and this led to a professional reconversion to this field. During this period he resumed university studies in the field of software engineering and upon completion of this, he commenced a new career in web development, which remains as his main occupation today.

Nicolas' other great interest lies in investing in the stock market and it has taken him 12 years to experiment with and develop effective investment methods. He now shares his findings in his first book, Le Guide de l'investisseur en Bourse qui Veut Décoller, translated in English as The Ultimate Guide for Successful Stock Investor: How to Smartly Deal With Markets to Get Rich.

In his spare time, Nicolas enjoys all sorts of sports, including running, judo and cycling. He was previously an experienced glider pilot, gaining some 130 hours in solo flight.

Nicolas is also passionate about new technologies and finding solutions to the problems of everyday life. In particular, helping people who are experiencing difficulties motivate him greatly.

Books

Betting Games Demystified: How To Bet On Games and Win: An Introduction to Games Betting and How To Create A Winning Strategy

The ultimate guide for successful stock investor: how to smartly deal with markets to get rich?

www.ingramcontent.com/pod-product-compliance
Lightning Source LLC
Chambersburg PA
CBHW030019190526
45157CB00016B/3138